How To Win Your War Against Depression

Contents

Depression Treatment Without Side Effects

Since the end of the Second World War, the rates of depression around the world have soared. Depression is an illness that can destroy lives ad families. Many people try various forms of treatment before any improvement is realized. Many are not so lucky and end up paying the ultimate price. Drugs and medication are one way to treat depression. However there has been a lot of criticism in recent years over the amount of medication we are taking. Depression can be treated naturally and the natural approach should be attempted first if possible.

Getting good nights sleep is essential. Sleep and mood are closely linked. When we are tired we react to things differently than we do when we have had adequate rest. Remember to sleep well and regularly.

Caffeine and other stimulants should be avoided. They do give you temporary energy but have been known to deplete your serotonin levels. Low serotonin levels are a prime cause of depression.

Take a multi vitamin everyday. This is especially important if your lifestyle causes you to skip meals. Low vitamin deficiency has been linked to depression.

You may want to try getting in touch with your spiritual side. This can be done in a variety of ways. If you enjoy going to church, this is a good opportunity. You may want to look at prayer and meditation as well. You do not have to be overly religious to be spiritual. There are many ways to get there.

Finally, you may want to try getting more exercise. This doesn't mean marathon training. Start out slow and build up if you feel the need. Exercise helps release endorphins which make you feel more empowered. There is also the health benefits attached to more activity.

The natural approach may be effective. It can also have other positive influences on your overall health.

Depression Treatment: Natural Treatments

The natural approach isn't always the best or most effective. However, if the depression isn't severe and the person isn't suicidal or incapacitated, then it is recommended to at least give the natural way a chance.

There are many natural remedies that can be tried before trying drugs and medication. Some have tried that natural remedy known as St. John's wort. This has been known to improve the mood of some depression sufferers without any side effects.

Those that suffer from depression should avoid excessive alcohol intake. Alcohol is a depressant so it will slow your body down. It could react with your body's chemistry and make your condition worse. Alcohol is also a toxin that they body does not need.

Try to eat a well balances diet. Loss of vitamins and minerals are directly linked with depression. Make time to eat despite the type of lifestyle you have.

You may want to consider cognitive behavior therapy. This will help you refocus your thought and generate a more positive feeling. Your thoughts have a direct bearing on your mood. The more negative they are the more likely you are to become depressed.

If you lead a stressful lifestyle, then some stress management training could be for you. Stress can be the cause of all kinds of ailments, not only depression. Keeping your stress levels low and learning to deal with highly stressful situations can go a long way in helping your depression.

You may want to try helping others. Sometimes doing volunteer work and helping those less fortunate will help. It can be quite rewarding and can negate some of those negative thoughts about yourself.

If the natural approach does not work, you should not feel bad. It is fine to take medications if this is what will help. You can at least be pleased for giving the natural approach a try.

Depression Treatment: Helping Someone Else

If someone you love is suffering from depression, it is only natural to want to help. Family members can provide an incredible amount of support for someone suffering from this illness. However, you must know how to be effective. If not the family member could end up doing more harm than good.

The first thing you should do is read everything you can about depression and its treatments. Being forewarned is being forearmed. By making yourself knowledgeable, you can help make decisions when perhaps the loved one isn't in a fit state to do so. You should also read up on how your loved one will feel. Getting as much insight as possible as to what depression will do to this person will help you cope with the worst days.

You have to keep in mind that caring for a depressed person is very braining both physically and emotionally. You need to set aside time for yourself. You won't be any use to your loved one if you are tired and stressed out. In fact you may make things worse. Talk about what you are going through with someone who understand or even join a support group. Take some time to enjoy yourself as well. Don't let your loved ones depression takes over your life as well.

Depressed people do need lots of love and support. You don't want to smother them but you need to be there when they need it most. Knowing they can rely on you will help them get through some of the darkest moments.

Don't deny your own feelings. There will be times when you're feeling angry and frustrated. You need a support network to help vent these feelings out. A good friend or a support group again can be a great source of comfort. Keeping your feelings bottled up can lead to your own illness.

Depression Treatment: Talking Therapies

Dealing with depression is difficult and draining. It puts stress and strain on the life of the depressed person as well as those close to him or her. Many types of therapies may have to be tried and tested before any improvement is seen. One such possibility is talk therapy.

Talking therapies can be of a great help when it comes to treating depression. It involved various types of counseling with a psychologist, Psychiatrist or therapist. Talking therapies allow the depressed person to get their feelings out. They also allow for the two people to work together to try to find the root cause for their depression.

Talking therapies do vary but most involve the same key elements. First there is the listening session. The therapist listens to the person's problems. Over time the person develops a relationship with the therapist where they feel they are understood. Next there is the emotional release. This is helpful but cannot be done to often. Letting the emotions out too often can have the opposite effect and lead to further depression. Next comes the advice and guidance. The patient may be able to seek the answers on their own through session and homework. Finally, there is information provided. They are giving information in small bits but as progress is made it can be increased. Depressed people can sometimes have poor concentration and memories so information is given carefully.

Talking therapies can be very effective in treating depression but they do take time. Several sessions may be required and the patient's family may have to be involved. Talking therapies can help mild to moderate depression greatly; however severe cases of depression will usually need a combination of talk and medication.

Depression Treatment: ECT Therapies

Today we know more about depression than ever before. WE have more treatment methods and medications to help people get through this illness and function as normally as possible. Depression is a horrible illness and unfortunately it can take a long time before any improvement is seen. Most therapies and medications take a significant amount of time to work effectively. With all of the therapies that are available there are still a small percentage of people that seem beyond the reach of conventional therapy. For those that nothing else seems to work there is ECT therapy.

Giving ECT therapy isn't a decision to take lightly. It is usually only given when all other avenues have failed. It is also only used for people who are suffering from the most severe forms of depression. Those that are suicidal and those that completely incapacitated by their depression are those that are considered for ECT therapy.

When a patient received ECT treatment, electrical impulses are sent into the brain. This then causes a small seizure to take place. The patient is under heavy sedation while this happens and awakens with no memory of what has happened. Sometimes they awake confused and feeling ill. However, the memory loss is usually temporary.

ECT is repeated 6-12 times at intervals separated by a few weeks. Many patients do feel an improvement after just a few sessions. It is believed that the electrical impulses change the pattern in the brain. ECT has worked on several people and most of the time the effects are temporary.

ECT therapy is given only when absolutely necessary. When it is though that the depression symptoms need to be taken away immediately, then ECT is a possibility.

Taking Manic Depression Seriously

The Symptoms Of Manic Depression

An extremely common and unfortunately the worst type of depression is the manic form. A person suffers from repeated mood swings and has frequent highs and lows. Behavior takes on an erratic form, and moods can change from happy to sad within seconds. Some people think that Pre menstrual syndrome could be the cause or even stress, but this is not so.

A person can get annoyed over the slightest incident and sometimes it could be something quite unimportant like the flavor of ice cream. Anger and irritability ensue leading to an unpleasant display of words. All this can be a symptom of manic depression. Unfortunately, it could last for a week, and is not limited to just one day.

When a person is experiencing a low feeling, it could be equated with real depression. There are so many negative feelings that go through a person's mind like the inability to enjoy life and people, feelings of hopelessness and guilt, feelings that no one cares for them, panic attacks and acute negativism. Therapists feel that if this persists for over a week, a person can be labeled as manic depressive.

Treatment For Manic Depression

Manic depression is very common and can be severe, but the good news is that it can be treated. It is not necessary to worry about it, but see that the person is in touch with the therapist who can guide him with correct treatment and medication in the right amount. Regular visits are a must, so the person can interact and discuss all his feelings which he may not be able to do with family and friends.

It is possible to get good relief through natural forms of treatment, and this can be looked into as possible help for the individual, but for permanent relief, it is best to consult a cognitive behavior therapist who has the experience in dealing with manic depression and all problems related to the mind. He will be able to diagnose your condition and go deeply into your past and present behavior and find the necessary link to your actions and behavior. He is better equipped to deal

How To Win Your War Against Depression

with the situation, and will prescribe the necessary medication if he feels you need it – regular visits to him will give you a confidence boost and enable you to open up. With his experience in dealing with cases like yours, he will be able to give you the pros and cons of the treatment and advise you on what treatment is best for you. You need to remember that each individual is different, and what may be suitable for someone else may not be suitable for you. So, all you need to do is seek the best therapist in the field and get the help you need.

Natural Treatment For Depression

There are many natural methods that can be used to relieve depression – one of them is the relaxation technique – this is known to treat the visible symptoms that affect you. By relaxing, you can get your heart rate to a normal level, and you will be able to regain your focus and be able to concentrate. It can also help to reduce your blood pressure and eliminate dark thoughts that lead to depression.

You can try this natural relaxation treatment at home which will help you to eliminate anxious thoughts and de-stress yourself. You will also find that you have an increased burst of energy and the relaxing methods will help to improve your sleep and thus enable you to deal with your day to day affairs in a calm and controlled manner.

Natural Methods Using Muscle Relaxation Techniques

The natural method shows you how to relax your muscles in order to relieve tension in your entire body. This method has been around for more than 50 years. When you are in a depressed state of mind, it affects your relationship with those who are close to you – by relaxing your muscles, it helps to relieve the tension and thus your mind becomes clear and focused and you will be able to relate better to those around you.

By using this method of relaxation, your muscles are tightened, and to reach your goal, you need to practice. As your body gets less tense, your mind improves and you will be able to focus and concentrate and you will find that you are less stressed out and anxious. You could go for classes, or go on the internet – also watch TV and get as many tips as you can. If you need therapy, the combination of the two will do wonders for your state of mind while improving your bodily functions.

A very important feature of this natural method is the fact that it must be done on a regular basis and not in fits and starts if it is to be helpful. A daily program should be inculcated and should be kept up. Along with this program, you can add other things like meditation, which is known to clear your mind and fill it with peaceful and soothing thoughts. This will help you to relax. Also

How To Win Your War Against Depression

another form of relaxation is yoga, which is also good for the body and mind, as it soothes you, takes the stress out of your system and helps you to focus on positive thoughts.

Regular practice is the key, and this can help anyone, not necessarily only those who are suffering from depression. So, go ahead and get a start on your goal towards a positive and stress free life.

<u>Major Depression – Just Don't Bother Me!</u>

Depression – Both Mild And Severe

There are various forms of depression, some of them are mild and some of them can be very severe and even border on suicidal thoughts. Mild depression can take different forms like overeating or not wanting to meet people or friends, whereas major depression can put a hold on one's life – there seems to be no purpose or joy in life – in fact, there is the desire to stay in bed and not get out of the house.

Commercials on TV show persons suffering from major depression as listlessly looking out of the window, and when a wife speaks to the person, he is completely phased out, and seems to be in a dark world of his own.

The Symptoms Of Major Depression

There are so many things in life that can be destroyed by major depression. You do not have confidence in yourself, and this leads to withdrawing from the public and society in general. You become anti-social, and you keep family away thereby destroying relationships. Violence is a part of this depression. If you do not feel like eating, this could affect your physical well being.

Major depressive order is the term used for Major Depression. When you are aware of symptoms occurring on a daily basis like sleeplessness, a feeling of worthlessness and a lack of confidence, tiredness and being unable to make decisions even in little matters, and when these symptoms happen for 2 weeks at a stretch, then you know that you are going through major depression.

There are also negative thoughts about oneself and differences in moods and attitudes – for instance, a person may not want to associate with anyone and is basically not interested in the things he took part in previously. There is a general feeling of apathy and listlessness that reflects a negative state of mind.

How To Win Your War Against Depression

The most important symptom to look for is when a person has thoughts of taking his life when a feeling of hopelessness sets in. This is the time that you need to take stock of the situation, particularly with a loved one who needs your help, as the person may not be aware of the situation he is in, and in this case, he desperately needs help.

There is no need to despair, as there is help available and with the correct treatment a person can be cured. Extreme cases will have to be put on medication along with various forms of treatment. Anti-depressants will help in calming the person down, and once that is achieved, he can go on to different types of treatment. The main thing is to seek a specialized therapist who will make the correct diagnosis, evaluate the person's requirements, as each person's needs vary, and put him on the road to recovery.

Getting Anxious Over Anxiety Depression?

Causes Of Anxiety Depression

So many people put an extra strain on themselves by getting into tasks that they take upon themselves, and this naturally leads to stress. It is not only a strain on the body but it affects the mind as well – in severe cases it could lead to a nervous break down. Again, there are others who are hyper active and feel the need to get things done on time and this takes a toll on their health, both mentally and physically. For such people, there is help that they can seek and they can avail of this treatment for anxiety depression.

People who are stressed out because of undertaking a whole bunch of activities which they find difficult to cope with display certain nervousness and behavior that is erratic – they indulge in mood swings as pressure builds up. They need to relax more frequently and face things in a composed manner in order to retain their sanity.

In order to treat yourself, you need to make a self analysis of your thoughts and behavior, so that you can consult with a therapist and get yourself the right cure.

Different Types Of Depression

There are various types of depression – Manic and Cyclothemia are similar because the person has mood swings – they can experience highs and lows frequently. Dysthimia is not as severe, but needs to be treated as soon as possible. Then there is Postpartum depression which involves extreme stress during childbirth and the fear of taking care of a new baby – this also needs to be taken care of at once. There is a depression that occurs during the change of seasons, particularly in Winter – moods change and become melancholy and feelings of irritation and anger are known to haunt a person.

The most common type of depression is Anxiety Depression. While it is normal to worry about every day things, to be continually worrying over anything that happens needs to be dealt with by visiting a therapist.

How To Win Your War Against Depression

GAD is known as a Generalized Anxiety Disorder where a person displays a greater sense of paranoia and is greatly stressed out for no known cause – there are also symptoms that occur like sleeplessness , inability to concentrate and focus, inertia, but the good news is that there is treatment available and when you recognize these symptoms, you should visit a therapist who will diagnose your symptoms and treat it accordingly. Medication may be prescribed, which will help to calm your nerves, so with the right therapist and medication you will be on the road to recovery.

Medication As Treatment

Sometimes doctors prescribe medication for severe forms of depression, but there are many cases where the person does not respond and so medication is not for everyone, but depends on the individual case. Doctors do not prescribe medication except as a last resort, when a person is severely depressed and has thoughts of taking his life, or if a person is delusional and could become violent, and again, if depression returns frequently thus impinging on a person's life.

Medication for depression may be given if everything else has been tried and proved futile, or if a person has not responded to psychotherapy and is violent and cannot be controlled. Doctors will only go for medication after intensive probing into the causes that have resulted in depression – for instance, they will delve into the past and present life of the person, so that they can decide on the best form of treatment. If all else fails, then they will prescribe medication.

Different Types Of Medication

There are various types of medication that may be prescribed – the usual ones are serotonin or benzodiazepine tranquilizers or tricyclics. These medications are prescribed because the quantity of chemicals in the brain is not correct and this results in the neurotransmitters being dysfunctional, which in turn produces a great deal of worry and stress in the person.

There are any number of anti-depressants and tranquilizers that are used to treat a person. But the doctor has to consider each individual's capacity to absorb the medication and decide whether it is suitable. Many medications have unpleasant side effects and therefore it is not advisable to continue them – also some medicines are habit forming, and like any harsh drug, will need to be slowly withdrawn. These drugs are very strong and the doctor will only prescribe them when absolutely necessary.

There are certain drugs that do not have the same effect as anti-depressants – in other words, they do not attack the same chemicals, but they have an effect on the moods and stabilize them.

How To Win Your War Against Depression

Not everyone can take medication, especially if a person is pregnant or if a person is on other medication, then the two cannot mix. On the other hand, there are certain medications that can be safely taken together. Your doctor will advise you as to what is appropriate. As far as possible , it is better to treat the root of the problem with careful counseling, and only if there is no response and the condition worsens, can one resort to medication. As medications for depression are very strong with side effects, many people find it tedious to continue and so give it up. When the condition recurs, they have no option but to go back on medication. Whatever you decide, it is best to consult your doctor and take his expert advice.

Depression

The Different Forms Of Depression

It is extremely difficult to recognize the difference between everyday stresses and anxieties, and actual depression. There are various forms of depression and the underlying causes may go back to the past and a person's childhood. You need to assess your emotions which may include stress, worry and anxiety, and if you feel that it is a little too frequent, then maybe it would be a good idea to do a depression test. Each person reacts differently, and no two cases are identical. Identifying your emotions will give you an insight as to whether you should see your doctor, particularly if you have panic attacks frequently. A depression test will help you to decide whether it is necessary to visit your doctor who will be able to refer you to a physiotherapist so that you will get the help you need.

A Depression Test

By taking a depression test, you will be able to identify your symptoms, because many people do not know that their feelings and thoughts are bordering on the morbid and that they are in a state of depression. Their life is slowly becoming different and it could be due to a variety of factors.

The person who is experiencing depression can take a depression test, or the near and dear ones, as also friends who are unable to discover whether their loved one is actually in a state of depression or not. The test is merely to see whether these symptoms occur for more than 2 weeks, and if they do, then it is a sure sign that you may need to see your doctor who will be able to help you.

The symptoms that you need to look out for are:

Morbid thoughts that come out of nowhere, like feeling that your life is worthless and that nobody cares whether you are around or not, the inability to make decisions, procrastination, feelings of shame, unable to enjoy yourself in a crowd or even with friends, lack of exercising, dislike of being with family, loss of appetite, sleeping too much or not at all, listlessness. If these

How To Win Your War Against Depression

feelings are what you are going through, then a depression test will definitely help you to identify your problem and seek the help you need.

Apart from affecting your mind, depression can affect your physical well being too as well as your interaction with close friends and relatives. Once you have taken a depression test, the next thing to do is to monitor your mood swings, and make a note of your varying changes in behavioral patterns. This could be shown to your doctor who will be able to guide you, and in any case this self analysis is a therapy for your own well being.

Causes Of Depression

Medical Research On Depression

There have been innumerable studies on depression, and various theories have been put forward as to why people fall into a depressed state of mind. The general opinion that has been shared by the medical faculties is that there are a variety of causes that cause depression and it cannot be attributed to any one factor. Research is still going on, and great headway has been made over the years.

Many doctors feel that depression could surface as a result of genes inherited. They feel that certain traits are bound to appear in forthcoming generations. Also, these genes could adversely interfere with the serotonin that the brain produces. Finally, the only conclusion that medical researches can arrive at is that a variety of factors can cause depression, and while eliminating these factors one by one, the person can be treated successfully.

Childhood Experiences

Doctors usually will go deeply into a person's childhood and try and find out factors that could inhibit a person. For instance, if a person has had uncomfortable experiences in the physical or sexual sphere, this could have a direct impact on a person's emotional well being. The future could seem bleak and a sense of worthlessness prevails. Also the person is inhibited socially and tends to isolate himself.

Depression could also be a biological factor. One has to bear in mind that there are chemicals in the brain that help us to guard against danger – our reflexes are able to help us to protect ourselves, but if there is a chemical imbalance, then we cannot react as quickly. Also, keeping feelings dormant only serves to bring out morbid thoughts and feelings and an inability to handle any form of anxiety or stress.

Medical Conditions And Drugs As A Cause Of Depression

There are certain ailments like hyperthyroidism that can seriously affect a person's ability to handle situations regarding a job loss or the death of a loved one. Attacks of panic frequently occur, as the person is unable to handle any emotional blow. Handling pain effectively can be difficult under these circumstances.

Drugs like cocaine can have a devastating effect on the brain, and can damage the brain cells, cause attacks of paranoia and produce imbalance, so that the person is in a constant state of nervousness and fear.

The human race is complicated and in order to deal with depression effectively, it is very important to analyze the root of the problem, which may go far back to one's childhood experiences or to certain shocks like the loss of a job or a loved one, traumatic changes in one's life as a result of these devastating losses – all these need to be focused upon and dealt with accordingly, and with the help of medication and treatment available, you will be on the road to recovery.

Clinical Depression Symptoms

Identifying Clinical Depression

The reason it is so difficult to diagnose a person suffering from clinical depression is because a person does not behave in an abnormal manner, like maintaining long silences or not getting ready for the day. In fact, the person may not know that they are depressed, and so it is even more difficult for doctors to pinpoint that a person is in fact suffering from depression.

The main focus that doctors rely upon is to identify the cause. The brain holds the key as it sends messages through neurotransmitters which are in turn controlled by chemicals like Serotonin and Dopamine. These chemicals need to be produced in certain quantities – when this doesn't happen, then the neurotransmitters cannot work. This produces a chain reaction which affects a person's thought processes and finally depression sets in. In order to treat a person successfully, it is important to find out behavioral patterns, both past and present. Maybe the person does not want to meet people socially which he was doing in the past.

There could also be physical symptoms like a rise in blood pressure or a weight change.

Feelings Of Hopelessness

Other symptoms can affect the mind leading to feelings of hopelessness. Dark and negative thoughts frequent the mind and this exhibits itself in a person's behavior. They feel that life is not worth living. Everything seems worthless and there seems no joy, and there is nothing worthy to anticipate. They dwell on the errors they have committed and seem incapable of leading a normal life. If you are experiencing any of these feelings, then you are probably going through a bad phase of depression, but there is always help for you.

Sometimes a person can behave in a manner that exhibits fear and worry by dissolving into tears or being overly anxious. They may not want to join in any group functions or attend parties, and even if they do, they tend to withdraw into themselves and remain aloof. Or they may refuse to be drawn into any topic as they prefer to be by themselves. Talking tires them, and they feel their energy being depleted.

How To Win Your War Against Depression

There are times when clinical depression manifests itself in very obvious signs like mania, and this definitely requires immediate treatment. If it is not treated, it could only worsen the situation and be a cause for alarm. If your mind is filled with dark and negative thoughts, and you blame yourself for all your mistakes, and do not want to spend time with those who are close to you like your own kith and kin and other friends, and if your body has undergone a change – maybe weight loss or if you suddenly have a medical condition, then you should visit your physician who will refer you to the right doctor who can evaluate your needs and help you accordingly.

Chronic Depression

Various Forms Of Treatment For Chronic Depression

This form of depression lasts for a while, maybe even 2 years, and a person experiences this on and off. It doesn't really go away completely but keeps coming back, even though it may not be in a severe form.

Doctors and therapists try different methods of treatment like group therapy and counseling before putting a person on to medication. Some people respond and can thus avoid anti-depressants and medication, but if all else fails, the only option is to go for medication which is not really a permanent solution.

Chronic Depression Known As Dysthymia

Dysthymia which is the form of chronic depression is not a severe illness, and does not keep you dysfunctional, but it exhibits itself in different forms, mainly lack of concentration, hopeless feelings regarding life, tendencies of taking one's life and a complete lack of confidence. These feelings remain with a person daily and may last for long periods of time, even years. Although you can go on with your life, these sad feelings cramp you and make you feel that your life is worthless.

Dysthymia can occur at any stage of a person's life – it is not restricted to any particular age group – it could affect both young and old alike. Since there are no visible symptoms that affect bodily functions, and a person is able to discharge his duties, it is extremely difficult to pinpoint. But, this condition cannot be neglected, as it will not go away by itself, so treatment has to be sought to set the condition right.

If the treatment is sought early, it will arrest the condition and prevent it from escalating into something so severe that it will have to be treated with anti-depressants and drugs which are very strong and may need to be continued almost permanently. Many doctors have come across cases that do not respond to treatment, but do not lose heart, as there are various other forms of treatment, and you can consult your physician who will be able to recommend a good therapist who will administer the care that you require.

How To Win Your War Against Depression

The most important thing is to recognize that you are feeling low and that you do not seem to enjoy life, or tend to shy away from people because of a lack of confidence. You also need to assess the length of time that you have been feeling this way, and the symptoms that seem to be surfacing that is preventing you from leading a full life. Once this has been identified, then you can go on to the next step which is seeking the necessary help,

The Truth About Postpartum Depression

The Views Of Tom Cruise And Brooke Shields

Tom Cruise, while talking on the Today Show expressed his views on Postpartum depression and totally disagreed with Brooke Shield's decision to take medication instead of exploring natural methods which are healthy like exercise. Many people don't realize the intricacies of depression and the way to treat it.

Postpartum Depression is an illness that needs to be studied so as you can be aware of the dangers and you can help other people who are suffering. Pregnancy is a difficult period and the thought of handling a new baby and the responsibilities involved in bringing up the child is something that can be frightening to a person who is not strong willed. Even if a person avoids alcohol and smoking, vigorous exercise and a stressful life, bad and negative thoughts can affect the baby growing inside.

Reasons For Postpartum Depression

Although people have discovered the causes of Postpartum depression and have taken steps to eliminate it either through medication or counseling as in the case of Brooke Shields, it can still be prevented. A new mother is particularly susceptible, and Postpartum depression is very much like depression.

Childbirth can be stressful both physically and mentally – the body undergoes hormonal changes and this can be uncomfortable, while affecting a person's moods. This is a leading cause of Postpartum depression. Many mothers who have been unwilling to go through the process of childbirth and look upon it with fear are most likely to fall into Postpartum depression. Instead of being joyful at the prospect of having a new baby and being a mother, they see it as something that will cause them strain, pain and stress.

If a person is a victim of Postpartum depression, it is absolutely necessary to visit a therapist, as the child can be hurt because the mother has angry feelings towards the child and feels that the child is the cause of all her problems like being overweight and unattractive. It is absolutely

How To Win Your War Against Depression

essential to seek a good therapist who will have counseling sessions with the person, and if all else fails, the therapist will put her on medication depending on the severity of the illness. This is something that cannot be ignored, as Postpartum depression can be the root cause of even murder. The mother is unaware of what is taking place in her head and feels the child is responsible for all her physical and mental pain. In order to avoid a tragedy, it is best to seek out good medical advice, be in touch with a therapist who will guide you and help you to move forward with medication if necessary.

What Is Bipolar Depression?

Bipolar depression is the term used to refer to the disorder characterized by major swings in a person's mood. At one moment he may feel elated and confident, and shortly afterwards the feeling abruptly changes to one of defeat and failure. The experience is similar to those occasions when one's feelings of well-being and happiness turn sour at a sudden turn of events or circumstances. The difference is that in bipolar depression, these mood swings occur regularly, sometimes even occurring daily, and without any rhyme, reason or regard to circumstance.

The high points as well as the low points during the mood swings in bipolar depression do approach the extreme ends of the mood spectrum and can often lead to irrational behavior. People diagnosed correctly with bipolar depression often experience euphoric highs and may actually believe they are incapable of defeat or injury. There may be occasions when bipolar persons gamble uncontrollably or decide to go on a shopping spree without any regard for their financial state or the probability of dire consequences that may follow. As the euphoria swings swiftly to a severely depressed state, the memory of a just-ended and short-lived euphoria haunts him and intensifies the depression even more. While such extreme examples are not generally common, lesser degrees of euphoria and sudden depression occurring regularly in an alternating fashion can still be quite confusing and definitely exhausting. There is an endless array of possibilities towards a path of difficulties in the personal and family life.

A person suffering from bipolar depression in the workplace may bring potentially harmful consequences. Decisions made rashly during a period of extreme highs may very well result in serious damages to the company or his co-workers. Some of those who suffer from bipolar depression sometimes become hyperactive and believe they are omnipotent and can do no wrong.

Bipolar depression can also be brought about through substance abuse. A diagnosis of bipolar depression has become very common among drug users and researchers are studying the seeming relation between drug abuse and the bipolar or the manic depression. It is observed that once a person is diagnosed with this ailment due to drug abuse, it is common that patients have to deal with it through the rest of his life.

How To Win Your War Against Depression

Once a valid and proper diagnosis of bipolar depression is made, a person will have to manage the condition for rest of his life. Children sometimes do develop bipolar depression but the condition is often misdiagnosed as attention deficit hyperactivity disorder(ADHD) or even simple hyperactivity.

While the disorder is a complex medical issue, the present treatment for bipolar depression generally does help those who suffer from it. After medical attention, their lives get back to normal. The regimen of treatment normally requires medication to reduce the severity of the moods, and some form of psychotherapy to inform the person suffering from bipolar depression of the manifestations of the disorder and instruct him how to recognize its onset. As research on bipolar depression goes further, there is hope that future developments will lead to better and more effective treatments.

Depression Treatment: How To Avoid Side Effects

Depression is a difficult condition to conquer. It leaves some sufferers completely useless and without hope for the future. Some become housebound while others end up taking their own lives. Depression affects different people in different ways. Some are fine for a time and then slip into their depressed state. Others experience a more chronic version of the condition.

Depression can be treated. However it may take a variety of therapies. These therapies do take time to work. Some want to stay away from drug treatments. While they can be quite effective they can leave you with many side effects. Depression can be treated naturally and it is usually the first course of action. In this article, we will look at ways to naturally treat depression.

Getting good nights sleep is essential. Sleep and mood are closely linked. When we are tired we react to things differently than we do when we have had adequate rest. Remember to sleep well and regularly.

Caffeine and other stimulants should be avoided. They do give you temporary energy but have been known to deplete your serotonin levels. Low serotonin levels are a prime cause of depression.

Take a multi vitamin everyday. This is especially important if your lifestyle causes you to skip meals. Low vitamin deficiency has been linked to depression.

You may want to try getting in touch with your spiritual side. This can be done in a variety of ways. If you enjoy going to church, this is a good opportunity. You may want to look at prayer and meditation as well. You do not have to be overly religious to be spiritual. There are many ways to get there.

Finally, you may want to try getting more exercise. This doesn't mean marathon training. Start out slow and build up if you feel the need. Exercise helps release endorphins which make you feel more empowered. There is also the health benefits attached to more activity.

Treating depression can be difficult. Many are reluctant to try drug therapies due to their

How To Win Your War Against Depression

massive side effects. Depression can be treated naturally. A natural approach is less stressful on the body and can provide other health benefits. Try treating depression the natural way first. The other methods will still be there if it fails.

Depression Treatment: ECT Therapies

Today we know more about depression than ever before. WE have more treatment methods and medications to help people get through this illness and function as normally as possible. Depression is a horrible illness and unfortunately it can take a long time before any improvement is seen. Most therapies and medications take a significant amount of time to work effectively. With all of the therapies that are available there are still a small percentage of people that seem beyond the reach of conventional therapy. For those that nothing else seems to work there is ECT therapy.

Giving ECT therapy isn't a decision to take lightly. It is usually only given when all other avenues have failed. It is also only used for people who are suffering from the most severe forms of depression. Those that are suicidal and those that completely incapacitated by their depression are those that are considered for ECT therapy.

When a patient received ECT treatment, electrical impulses are sent into the brain. This then causes a small seizure to take place. The patient is under heavy sedation while this happens and awakens with no memory of what has happened. Sometimes they awake confused and feeling ill. However, the memory loss is usually temporary.

ECT is repeated 6-12 times at intervals separated by a few weeks. Many patients do feel an improvement after just a few sessions. It is believed that the electrical impulses change the pattern in the brain. ECT has worked on several people and most of the time the effects are temporary.

ECT therapy is given only when absolutely necessary. When it is though that the depression symptoms need to be taken away immediately, then ECT is a possibility.

Depression is an illness that can destroy people, families and relationships. The illness leaves people feeling hopeless and in some cases renders them completely useless. Today, we have many ways to treat depression. Talk therapies, natural therapies and medications are some of the most common. However, when all of these avenues fail, then ECT is considered. ECT is quite controversial. It carries with it an element of danger but has worked for several people who

How To Win Your War Against Depression

had been suffering from severe depression. ECT can have side effects but can also help those that no other therapy seems to help.

Depression Treatment: Treating It Naturally

Living with depression presents challenging circumstances. The dark moods one can experience can make just functioning seem impossible. Depression can have a wide variety of results. It can be treated, in many cases with 100% success. It can also have the worst outcome, involving someone taking their own life. Today, we are under constant pressure to stay away from drugs. Especially when it comes to treating mental illnesses. Medications do have their time and place, but it might be best to try to treat depression through natural means first.

There are many natural remedies that can be tried before trying drugs and medication. Some have tried that natural remedy known as St. John's wort. This has been known to improve the mood of some depression sufferers without any side effects.

Those that suffer from depression should avoid excessive alcohol intake. Alcohol is a depressant so it will slow your body down. It could react with your body's chemistry and make your condition worse. Alcohol is also a toxin that they body does not need.

Try to eat a well balances diet. Loss of vitamins and minerals are directly linked with depression. Make time to eat despite the type of lifestyle you have.

You may want to consider cognitive behavior therapy. This will help you refocus your thought and generate a more positive feeling. Your thoughts have a direct bearing on your mood. The more negative they are the more likely you are to become depressed.

If you lead a stressful lifestyle, then some stress management training could be for you. Stress can be the cause of all kinds of ailments, not only depression. Keeping your stress levels low and learning to deal with highly stressful situations can go a long way in helping your depression.

You may want to try helping others. Sometimes doing volunteer work and helping those less fortunate will help. It can be quite rewarding and can negate some of those negative thoughts about yourself.

How To Win Your War Against Depression

Finally, if you need to take medication, don't feel like a failure. It may be that the natural way isn't going to work for you. Be satisfied that you gave it a go.

Depression can present many challenges to a person. They range of emotions they feel can leave them feeling helpless and useless. Some do get treatment while others grow worse with each passing day. When possible look to natural treatments. They will not give you side effects and will give your body other health benefits. However, if it doesn't work there is no shame in treating your depression with medication. Whatever works for you is the best course of action.

Depression Treatment: Recognizing Depression

Depression is caused by many factors. Two of those factors are stress and burn out. When we are stressed our body's react differently then when we are relaxed. It can lead to many types of illnesses one of which is depression. If the body is under too much stress for too long it will simply shut down. The person will simply cease to function in the same capacity.

It is impossible to avoid stress in our lives completely. We all are under pressure at one time or another. This can be healthy at times as well. However, constant stress will eventually have negative effects. In this article we will look at the signs of overstress and burn out. These can eventually lead to chronic depression.

People who are under constant stress may seem chronically fatigued, tired and run down. Stress depleted your energy sources and leaves your body feeling physically drained. This symptom is quite dangerous because it is directly linked to depression.

Sometimes people get angry at those making demands. We can all over react at some point or another but if they show excessive anger at the slightest request then this person may need a break.

Sometimes people will get increasingly self critical. They may be angry at themselves for letting things pile up or for giving into everyone's demands. Anger at ones self can be linked to depression so this is a sign that should raise some alarms.

Sometimes when people are under incredible stress and strain they feel like they are being besieged. They feel the world is out to get them and display feelings of extreme paranoia. Again, irrational thinking is also a sign of depression so keep a close eye on anyone that is displaying this behavior.

If people seem to be having frequent headaches or gastrointestinal problems then this is a sign they are under too much stress. This can lead to serious health problems if they don't slow down.

How To Win Your War Against Depression

Knowing when someone is under too much stress and strain can have an effect on depression. Stress is one of the leading causes and knowing the warning signs could make the difference between severe depression and coping with stress. If you or anyone you know are showing these symptoms then encourage them to seek help. The alternative could be far worse.

Depression Treatment: Helping Someone Else

Depression can destroy lives. One of the worst things in life is having to cope with a family member or loved one that is suffering from this condition. You want to be as supportive as possible but you also have your own needs to consider. Loved ones can provide some of the most essential treatment available. The support network that they can offer can have profound positive effects. In this article we will look at how you can help someone who is suffering from depression.

The first thing you should do is read everything you can about depression and its treatments. Being forewarned is being forearmed. By making yourself knowledgeable, you can help make decisions when perhaps the loved one isn't in a fit state to do so. You should also read up on how your loved one will feel. Getting as much insight as possible as to what depression will do to this person will help you cope with the worst days.

You have to keep in mind that caring for a depressed person is very braining both physically and emotionally. You need to set aside time for yourself. You won't be any use to your loved one if you are tired and stressed out. In fact you may make things worse. Talk about what you are going through with someone who understand or even join a support group. Take some time to enjoy yourself as well. Don't let your loved ones depression takes over your life as well.

Depressed people do need lots of love and support. You don't want to smother them but you need to be there when they need it most. Knowing they can rely on you will help them get through some of the darkest moments.

Don't deny your own feelings. There will be times when you're feeling angry and frustrated. You need a support network to help vent these feelings out. A good friend or a support group again can be a great source of comfort. Keeping your feelings bottled up can lead to your own illness.

Depression can affect more people than just the depressed person. Coping with loved ones depression can put a lot of strain on a family and a marriage. Familiar support can be a great source of comfort to a depressed person. The structure they can provide can be vital to their treatment. However, you have to know how to help. By giving love and support and taking care of yourself, you'll be able to best help your loved one.

Depression Treatment: Helping Someone Else More

If you're living with a person who suffers from depression, you naturally want to do all you can for them. You'll want to offer all of the support you can and aid in their recovery in any way possible. Depression can destroy families and lives if it is left untreated. However, what is important to remember is that you need to take time out for yourself as well. In this article we will look at further tips and advice on how to help a loved one who is depressed.

As a loved one of a depressed person, you'll need to be prepared for possible personality changes and changes of attitude. The person may not want to engage in activities like they used to. They may not respond to you sexually or emotionally. This does not mean that they do not love you anymore. It is simply the illness. Be patent and supportive. It is difficult when this happens but with time and patience it should pass.

Sometimes depressed people withdraw to a point where the simplest of tasks seems too much to bear. Thinks like paying bills, housework and shopping are too much for them to cope with. You may need to take over for a while and do these tasks for them. You have to keep in mind that this is an illness so all the help you can give will aid in their recovery.

Treatment is essential if the depressed person is ever going to recover. They may not want to go or they may forget there sessions or medications. You need to remind them and keep encouraging them to go. Without treatment they will not improve and may even get worse.

Depression tends to take hope away from people. They feel like there is never going to be any change and the future will not get any better. You need to remind them that there is hope and offer it in any way that you can.

You will experience feeling of anger. It is okay to let them know that you are angry with their illness but not with them. It is important to distinguish between the two. If they feel you angry with them it may aggravate their symptoms.

Finally, you must keep things in perspective. You will not cure their depression so don't fool yourself into thinking you can. Simply provide all of the support you can. Depression can have an impact on your life but it doesn't have to take it over.

Depression Treatment: Depression In The Workplace

One of the best ways of treating depression is knowing the signs. Depression can happen to anyone and knowing how to recognize it is the first step in treating them. There are quite a few cases of depression associated with the workplace. Those in highly stressful jobs or jobs that are not that desirable can be prone to workplace depression. In this article we will look at some of the signs displayed with workplace depression. We will look at how to recognize it and ways you can help.

Educating yourself about depression is the first step. If you have an employee that is suffering from depression, even if their condition is under control, they may not be your best worker. Look out for low productivity. Keep in mind that this isn't a character flaw, it is an illness.

Sometimes those that are depressed stop caring about their own safety. If you notice them taking a lot of unnecessary risks then this is a sign. If they seem highly accident prone this is another indicator.

Look out for frequent mood changes. They may go from anger to sadness and even become uncooperative.

You should look out for low morale. If the seem to be complaining about several aspects of their life then depression could be a definite possibility.

IF they seem to be constantly tired then this could be a cause for concern. Depression can cause chronic fatigue. If they seem tired all the time or constantly complain about feeling fatigued then you may want to be concerned.

If these employees seem to be absent a lot then again, this could be a sign of depression. Many will call in with colds and flu symptoms since no one will except calling in depressed.

Sometimes the depressed person will self medicate with drugs and alcohol. If this is apparent then there should be cause for concern. This problem needs to be dealt with quite urgently.

How To Win Your War Against Depression

Workplace depression does exist and can be treated. As an employer the first thing you need to do is learn to recognize the signs. Next you need to educate yourself about depression. Finally, you need to encourage your employee to seek help. These are some of the best ways an employer can fight workplace depression.

Depression Treatment: Depression In The Workplace, Continued

Depression can be quite a destructive illness. There is the stress and strain it can put on a family or relationship, as well as the loss of productivity it can cost in the workplace. Employers loose money due to depression. Money lost from employee accidents and absenteeism make it work an employers while to learn to spot the signs. An employer cannot treat or cure depression but there are things that they can do to help. In this article we will look further into how to spot workplace depression and what you can do to help.

Look for signs of decreased productivity. This can be especially worrying if the person was once a good worker and their productivity levels start declining. There could be an underlying cause and depression is a possibility.

Those that are depressed quite often ignore the warnings about stress. This can cause the symptoms to manifest is a physical way. If you have an employee that is constantly complaining about aches and pains then this is a sign that depression could be the cause.

Try speaking to this employee. You need to let them know that you expect them to be productive. However, let them know that you notice the changes and are concerned. Don't make them feel like their job is in jeopardy. This could make things worse. If there are any employees assistance programs then try to encourage the employee to use them. This could be a first step on the road to their recovery.

You need to also set some clear guidelines about what you expect from the employee. Let them know the company policy toward depression related illnesses and what they are entitled to.

Make sure the employee knows that everything is confidential. Not even you are entitled to know what is discussed in sessions. Try to encourage them to seek treatment for their depression. If left untreated some serious consequences could arise.

If the employee does seek treatment you may have to allow for a more flexible work schedule. You will get the time back eventually with increased productivity. Severe depression can bring serious consequences. Any threats of suicide should not be taken lightly. Report it immediately so they can be referred. They will thank you for it later.

Depression Treatment: Talking Therapies

Depression is one of the most destructive illnesses we have. Since the second world war the levels of depression have sky rocketed. Depression can destroy families, relationships and result in lost money. Employers every year loose money through absent employees and accidents brought on by depression.

Treating depression is quite varied. Many try natural therapies while others opt for medications. There are literally hundreds of things that can be tried. Quite often the depressed person will have to try several therapies or a combination before they find the correct one. In this article, we will look at some of the different types of therapies out there to help treat depression.

Talking therapies can be of a great help when it comes to treating depression. It involved various types of counseling with a psychologist, Psychiatrist or therapist. Talking therapies allow the depressed person to get their feelings out. They also allow for the two people to work together to try to find the root cause for their depression.

Talking therapies do vary but most involve the same key elements. First there is the listening session. The therapist listens to the person's problems. Over time the person develops a relationship with the therapist where they feel they are understood. Next there is the emotional release. This is helpful but cannot be done to often. Letting the emotions out too often can have the opposite effect and lead to further depression. Next comes the advice and guidance. The patient may be able to seek the answers on their own through session and homework. Finally, there is information provided. They are giving information in small bits but as progress is made it can be increased. Depressed people can sometimes have poor concentration and memories so information is given carefully.

Talking therapies can be very effective in treating depression but they do take time. Several sessions may be required and the patient's family may have to be involved. Talking therapies can help mild to moderate depression greatly; however severe cases of depression will usually need a combination of talk and medication.

Depression is a very serious condition. It puts a heavy stress and strain on the family and the workplace. It costs the country billions in lost work time and injury insurance claims. Many types of therapy are used to help deal with depression. Talk therapies can be quite helpful but do take time.

Depression Treatment: Light Therapies

Depression is something that can destroy lives. The life of the person suffering from the illness is off course affected but so to are the lives of the people close to him or her. Families and loved ones feel the strain almost as much as the sufferer. Other areas of life are vulnerable as well. Work can suffer and well as social contacts.

Fortunately, today we know much more about depression. The approach is an illness rather than a disorder. There are many types of treatments that can be used to treat depression. Sometimes several or a combination of treatments may be required before improvement is realized. In this article we will look at light therapy and what is has accomplished in treating depression.

Light has been shown to reduce the brain's level of melatonin. A chemical that can cause one to feel down and depressed. By sitting in front of a bright light for at least 4 hours a day, marked improvement has been seen in many depression patients.

Light therapy can be conducted using a light box. Many start to get depressed as the seasons change. The days start getting shorter and the weather gloomier. This reduces the amount of sunlight that we are exposed to naturally so our serotonin levels start to drop. This makes everyone feel a bit low but a person suffering from depression will feel a great deal worse. The light box requires the person to sit in front. They can carry on with an activity provided they stay within 2-3 feet of the box. The light then helps to replace the serotonin levels and helps reduce the chances of depression.

Light therapy has been proven effective in other areas as well. It has been shown to help sleep disorders as well as re-adjust our body clocks.

Depression is an illness that can destroy people and families. When one becomes seriously depressed they can cease to function normally. Everyone close to the depressed individual can be affected. Spouses can be forced to take care of their loved one while other members suffer along with them. Fortunately there are several types of therapies that can be tried. Light therapy has proven quite effective. By using light, the serotonin levels can start to climb back up and reduce the chances of increased depression.

Anxiety Depression

Some people seem to have personalities that just seem more prone to causing anxiousness. The problem is constant stress and anxiety can lead to anxiety depression. People who experience anxiety on a regular basis have been found to have some common traits. They include the following.

• Always striving for perfectionism
• Feeling like a failure when goals are not met
• Nervous
• Often feels guilty about what they did or did not do
• Doesn't like to hear any criticism about their self
• Displays obsessive traits
• Invents things to worry about

If your thoughts are always leading you to self-criticism, the result can be the development of anxiety depression. If you realize you have the anxiety prone personality, you can prevent a slide into depression. But even if you already have anxiety depression, you can learn to think differently.

Anxiety depression is often self induced. In other words, you're so hard on yourself that you never come out ahead in your thoughts. You want to be perfect and no one can achieve perfection. You want to be all things to all people in your life, and that's not possible either. But because of these feelings and thoughts, you're never satisfied with your efforts. So you begin to tell yourself that you're a failure or worthless.

People experience different levels of anxiety depression. For example, you can have a mild case that affects your attitude toward yourself, but doesn't interfere with your activities. You can also have a severe form of anxiety depression that drives you deeper and deeper into the well of dissatisfaction. Treatment options include both self help and recognized therapies such as cognitive and behavioral. But the key in any treatment is to change your self perspective.

How To Win Your War Against Depression

One of the common symptoms of anxiety depression is the belief you can't express yourself, because then people won't like you. That lack of self-esteem makes you always put yourself last. You also may have expectations that are way too high making success impossible. During treatment, you learn to set reasonable goals and then how to accept the results of your efforts in a positive manner.

Anxiety depression can be debilitating if left unchecked. You have to learn to like yourself first. Everyone has special talents and abilities including you. If you put your personal energy into taking advantage of those abilities rather than suppressing them, you'll be amazed at how quickly you can rise out of your depression. Thoughts can be self-defeating and act like a trap. Open the trap and let those negative thoughts out and you can look at life from a whole new perspective.

Bipolar Depression

Bipolar depression is just what the name implies. It's a disorder that involves major swings in mood. One day you may be happy and ready to take on the world, and the next day feeling as if you don't even want to get out of bed. It's a very difficult disorder which is confusing and fatiguing. The mood swings can even happen in the space of a single day. If you've ever had one of those days where you went from feeling happy and successful to feeling like a failure, then you have an idea of what it's like to have bipolar depression. But imagine the swings happening regularly in your life – maybe even every day.

Bipolar depression is about a lot more than moods though. The highs and lows can be very extreme. In fact, people with bipolar depression have often have euphoric highs which lead them to act irrationally. While feeling euphoria, the person may believe they are invincible. For example, a bipolar person may think they can't lose at the casino and gamble all the household money. Or the person may decide to go shopping and buys everything in sight without regard to fiscal responsibility.

It's not too difficult to imagine how a person with bipolar depression can bring about devastation for a family. On the opposite end of the euphoric state is the depressed state. The state of depression can follow quickly and is especially low because of the memory of the short lived euphoria. You go from top of the world to not wanting to even get out of bed. Of course, not everyone has such extreme swings, but even lesser states of euphoria and depression can be difficult and confusing.

When someone is bipolar and holds a job, it's not hard to imagine the potential consequences. Rash decisions made during the high period can be very harmful to the job. Some people with bipolar depression get hyperactive and think they can do anything whether or not they're qualified.

Bipolar depression can be brought on by substance abuse. Drug users are commonly diagnosed with bipolar depression and studies are researching whether the propensity for drug use and the manic or bipolar depression are related. Once you are diagnosed with bipolar depression, it will most likely have to be managed the rest of your life. Even children can

How To Win Your War Against Depression

develop bipolar depression though it's frequently misdiagnosed as hyperactivity or attention deficit disorder.

Bipolar depression is a complicated medical issue but treatment works well. Treatment usually includes medication to even out the moods and psychotherapy to teach the person how to be aware of the onset of the mood swings. As researchers continue to study the problem, it's fully expected that new treatments will be developed.

Childhood Depression

Childhood depression doesn't seem like it should exist, because the time of being a child should be filled with thoughts of family, school and friends and not worry and anxiety. Yet it's an increasing problem in our society for many reasons. First, children are subject to the same problems as adults simply because they're human. They suffer stress, have family problems and may be born with a predisposition towards depression due to genetics. Second, depression is now diagnosed correctly more often than it was in the past.

Childhood depression makes itself known in a number of ways. The child may experience frequent high and low emotional states. Children who are depressed often don't want to leave the house and play with friends. Another symptom is a change in school performance. If he or she once did well in school and then loses interest, it can be a sign the child is depressed. Another frequent symptom is a lack of interest in normal activities. Early intervention is important in order to prevent progression of the disorder.

Childhood depression can be treated. Parents who think their child may be depressed can take certain steps to re-engage the child in a number of ways. The first thing you should do is try to get your child interested in something. It can be a social or athletic activity or even certain toys. Another important step to take is getting your child to talk to you regularly, but be careful of responding with only criticism. Just like in adult depression, childhood depression means the child is having problems with self esteem. Your goal is to build up feelings of self-worth so coping mechanisms are stronger.

One of the important steps you can take for treating childhood depression is working with your child to develop appropriate responses to situations. Life is always going to have those moments when you have to overcome perceived failure or difficult situations. If you child doesn't know how to respond and only gets frustrated, then childhood depression can take hold.

When you decide your child is experiencing depression, you need to try and uncover any particular causes. For example, if he or she is having trouble at school then perhaps there's a problem between your child and another child. Or if your child suddenly withdraws for no apparent reason, then you might need to have your child work with a therapist to investigate

How To Win Your War Against Depression

possible emotional or sexual abuse (there will be other signs too obviously). Another common cause of childhood depression is an unsuspected learning disability.

Many children are not good at communicating what they're thinking or feeling. That means you have to make an extra effort to "interpret" the situation. There are many treatment options if the self-help treatments don't work. These treatments are similar to the ones used to treat adult depression.

Clinical Depression

Doctors have specific terms for medical issues and clinical depression is one of them. Medical research is always ongoing and the results of the research are published for the medical community. This is true for all medical conditions being studied. The goal is to find cause and cure by first identifying common symptoms. When you have clinical depression it simply means you fit the current definition of what medical science considers true depression.

Once you are diagnosed with clinical depression, a variety of treatment options become available. They include cognitive and behavior therapy, interpersonal therapy and medication. Some components of the therapy can be undertaken by you without a doctor. For example, you can learn to stop spiraling negative thoughts about your abilities and self-esteem. You can keep a journal or make yourself become more active. But for many people, their clinical depression must be treated by a doctor.

Doctors who treat clinical depression often combine medication with one or more of the other therapies. The goal is to keep the medication level as low as possible with eventual cessation. Cognitive therapy has proven to be quite effective as a depression treatment during controlled studies. With cognitive therapy, you learn to start loving yourself by changing your perceptions.

Interpersonal therapy involves counseling which focuses on the people or events involving other people that may have triggered your depression. It can also simply work to improve your self esteem so you have better interpersonal relationships.   Behavior therapy, on the other hand, helps you change your self-defeating behavior. You learn to enjoy doing some activities again. Behavior therapy is often used with cognitive therapy to treat clinical depression.

There are several medications commonly used in the treatment of clinical depression. They include selective serotonin reuptake inhibitors (SSRI) and tricyclics. Anti-depressant medications is almost always prescribed when someone indicates they have suicidal thoughts. In other situations, it may be prescribed for a short period of time to give a person a head start on cognitive and behavior therapy.

How To Win Your War Against Depression

Naturally, only medical doctors can prescribe medication for clinical depression. But there are different kinds of psychotherapists who offer the other treatment options. These include clinical psychologists and psychiatrists. Psychiatrists can prescribe medication and provide cognitive, behavior and group therapy. When you have mild depression, you can also utilize the services of a trained counselor.

Clinical depression is depression that fits the mold so to speak. You have all the signs and symptoms of depression as identified through medical research. All depression is treatable and there's no reason for anyone to feel alone or helpless. There are many different options for treatment and they all work. So if you suspect you are experiencing depression, it's important to get help right away.

All About Clinical Depression

Depression, a mental illness that is often characterized by prolonged periods of sadness and melancholy, experts from the field of psychiatry say.

But just because one person is moping around and just generally hating the world around him or her, doesn't mean that it's already depression, but if this kind of behavior, the feeling of emptiness, loss of self-worth and absolutely no hope for happiness just goes on and on, then, yes, that individual is very much, indeed, depressed.

Still, there are various types of depression, from Manic or Bipolar depression - characterized by sudden and extreme changes in one's mood wherein one minute he or she is in an elevated state of euphoria while the next minute (day or week) he or she is feeling to be in a personal hell, Postpartum depression - characterized by a prolonged sadness and a feeling of emptiness by a new mother wherein physical stress during child birth, an uncertain sense of responsibility towards the new born baby can be just some of the possible factors why some new mother go through this, Dysthimia - characterized by a slight similarity with depression, although this time, it's been proven to be a lot less severe, but of course with any case, should be treated immediately, Cyclothemia - characterized by a slight similarity with Manic or Bipolar depression wherein the individual suffering from this mental illness may occasionally suffer from severe changes in one's moods, Seasonal Affective Disorder - characterized by falling in a rut only during specific seasons (i.e. Winter, Spring, Summer or Fall) studies however, prove that more people actually fall in to a rut more during the WInter and Fall seasons and lastly, Mood swings, wherein a person's mood may shift from happy to sad to angry in just a short time.

Clinical depression however, or as some might call as 'major' depression, is actually the medical term for depression. Actually clinical depression is more of a disorder rather than an illness since it basically covers only those who are suffering from symptoms related to depression. Clinical depression is how doctors usually refer to "depression" when giving a diagnose of their patient. It's basically just a medical term.

However, in spite of being an actual disorder, Clinical depression may well be treated. Doctors are actually highly optimistic that their patients who are suffering from Clinical disorder will be

How To Win Your War Against Depression

well on their way towards good mental health as long as they treated as soon as they have been diagnosed with Clinical depression. Patients who have been seeking for treatments for Clinical depression have proven to be quite successful in their quest, given that 80 percent of actual Clinical depression patients have been treated and has somewhat found relief from their disorder.

For those who may be seeking some answers for their Clinical depression related questions, the depression section of the health center is highly recommended, as well as books on psychiatry and the internet - which can offer a lot of helpful information with regards to Clinical depression although self-medication/treatment is highly disapproved of. Clinical depression may not pose as much as a threat as the other types of depression, but it is best to leave it to the hands of professionals who can safely attend to and cure this disorder.

Helping Yourself With Depression Help

If you're currently feeling so out of it, totally out of your normal system and just basically hating and ignoring almost, always everything and anyone that comes along, try to get yourself checked by a psychiatrist because you those little mood swings and erratic Ally McBeal-ish behavior that you're trying to ignore for some long may actually be symptoms of depression. Act fast because if you do, it'll certainly be a lot harder for you to be able to have yourself cured from this illness, especially once self-delusion starts to kick in.

Actually start by hauling your depressed ass into the hospital and get yourself diagnosed by a reputable psychiatrist, one that'll actually help you with your depression concerns, answer all the possible questions that you may have when it comes to depression as well as provide you with the best available to depression treatment that'll make you give yourself some good-old, yet extremely effective depression help. All it needs is the right attitude.

After actually being honest with yourself when it comes to actually being a patient who is suffering from depression, quit turning yourself into a victim and find out from these various types of depression the actual one that you're suffering from: Manic or Bipolar depression - characterized by sudden and extreme changes in one's mood wherein one minute he or she is in an elevated state of euphoria while the next minute (day or week) he or she is feeling to be in a personal hell, Postpartum depression - characterized by a prolonged sadness and a feeling of emptiness by a new mother wherein physical stress during child birth, an uncertain sense of responsibility towards the new born baby can be just some of the possible factors why some new mother go through this, Dysthimia - characterized by a slight similarity with depression, although this time, it's been proven to be a lot less severe, but of course with any case, should be treated immediately, Cyclothemia - characterized by a slight similarity with Manic or Bipolar depression wherein the individual suffering from this mental illness may occasionally suffer from severe changes in one's moods, Seasonal Affective Disorder - characterized by falling in a rut only during specific seasons (i.e. Winter, Spring, Summer or Fall) studies however, prove that more people actually fall in to a rut more during the Winter and Fall seasons and lastly, Mood swings, wherein a person's mood may shift from happy to sad to angry in just a short time. But in spite of how scary or how daunting a task is the road towards a sound mental health is, depression help abounds and is just up to you if you're willing to take in some of that depression

How To Win Your War Against Depression

help, may it be from your family, friends, support group and mainly starting from yourself, there really is a lot of depression help to go around.

The old adage, slowly but surely greatly applies in trying to treat depression, as the patient continues taking the prescribed medicines for his/her depression treatment, as well as the corresponding therapy sessions with the cognitive behavior therapist, a patient being treated from depression needs all the support and depression help that he or she can get.

While being treated for depression, the patient as well as his or her family and other loved ones are advised to make realistic goals concerning depression wherein, to not assume that their depression can be easily treated in a snap. Depression help begins with trying to understand the patient's situation and continue on being patient as well as always extending your help because depression help is never easy nor is the depression treatment itself, which is why both patients and loved ones need to help each other out through every step of the way. Never set goals that are high above your reach, give yourself some depression help by not being too hard on yourself, believe that you are good and strong enough to achieve your goals but only one step at a time.

Depression Medications

Depression medications are serious business, because they're strong drugs that impact your brain functioning. They're not to be taken lightly and some are even addictive. There's a reason why all antidepressant medications are strictly controlled. They need to be taken only under the supervision of a doctor.

Not everyone wants to turn to depression medications for relief though. Each person must work with his or her doctor to determine which course of treatment is right for your situation. Some people try all other forms of treatment first while others begin a combined treatment of medication and another therapy. These other therapies can include group therapy, cognitive and behavioral therapy, and even self-help therapy to name a few.

So how do you know when taking one of the depression medications is the right choice? The first things most doctors will consider is how long your depression has been occurring and which therapies you have tried. Other factors in the decision to use depression medications include religious values, other medications currently being taken, pregnancy and propensity for drug dependency. As you can see, it may be a very complex decision to use depression medications.

In our society, we too frequently see drugs as a quick fix for everything that ails us. But even if you and your doctor decide to try drugs, they won't work instantly. There are no quick fixes for depression. You will probably have to take the medications for many months and it will take weeks before you notice a change in your depression disorder. In the meantime, you want to continue any other therapies currently being used to treat your depression.

One of the main considerations for deciding to use depression medications is the severity of the disorder. If you have bipolar condition or are depressed at least 2 hours every day, you have severe depression. If your depression is preventing you from working and creating other serious problems in your life, medication might be used in the beginning. The nice thing about medication is it can be stopped down the road. You can take it for the months you need it and then as other therapies work, or your depression abates, you can withdraw from the drugs.

How To Win Your War Against Depression

Treatments other than depression medications offer a change in thinking and lifestyle for the long term. Using medications is a short term solution except in the most severe cases. When you learn positive self-talk or positive thinking, they're techniques you can use anywhere.

When you use depression medications, it might be necessary to try more than one in order to get the best drug combination.   You also must be aware that most of them have side effects, but these side effects are different for everyone. That's another reason why you need constant doctor supervision.

Depression Test

Sometimes it can be difficult distinguishing between the normal emotional ups and downs that people experience as part of life and depression. But when you begin to suspect that you should feel much better than you do about yourself and your world, taking a depression test can provide important direction.

Depression does not have one form. It can take many different forms in terms of symptoms, and no two people are alike. But there are certain symptoms that frequently occur and can serve as measures of your emotional status. If nothing else, taking a depression test can help you decide if you need to see a doctor. Another benefit of utilizing a depression test as a barometer of your emotional state is that if you are experiencing depression, it may be hard for you to define your symptoms.

The depression test is merely a checklist of symptoms you identify as being applicable to your situation. It can be amazing how many people are actually unaware they have a mild case of depression or don't realize how much their life has changed due to depression. There are so many manifestations of depression that it's impossible to list them all.

The depression test can be used by the person who suspects they are experiencing depression or by family or friends who aren't sure how to recognize depression in someone they love. It's important to identify depression as early as possible, because depression will get worse. The general rule of thumb is to consider if you have experienced several of any of the following symptoms for longer than 2 weeks.

• Thoughts your life is spiraling out of control
• Believing your life is unimportant
• Convinced no one would miss you if you were to die
• Can't make any decisions – even small ones
• Don't anticipate anything at all as being enjoyable
• Feeling ashamed all the time
• Experiencing frequent and unexplained crying
• Can't enjoy being with friends or attending events
• Stopped exercising

How To Win Your War Against Depression

• Giving up things once enjoyed
• Avoiding people whenever possible
• Feeling alone all the time
• Doesn't enjoy being with family anymore
• Feeling like no one understands you
• Losing appetite
• Unable to sleep or sleeping too much
• Having no energy

The depression test can include many more symptoms, but this gives you a good idea of the kinds of things you would take into consideration. As you can tell from the list, depression affects a lot more than just your emotions. It can affect your body and your relationships too.

Once you take the depression test, the next step is to begin tracking the mood changes. By creating a mood diary, there's now something very tangible and quite convincing to show a doctor or therapist. It also provides you a clear picture of what's happening and that can be very therapeutic in itself.

Finding The Right Depression Medication

Always feeling under the weather? Always not in the mood to be around others and have a good time? If you're suffering from prolonged sadness for quite some time now, you should face these bouts of depression and get yourself diagnosed by a psychiatrist, they're doctors who can actually help you out with your problem. Not to mention the various depression treatments, as well as all sorts of depression medication that doctors prescribe to their depression patients.

Fortunately depression can now be cured, especially when diagnosed early, depressed individuals can actually be treated through therapy and depression medication, although it may be a bit costly, a person's good mental health is something that shouldn't be scrimped on. Cognitive behavioral talk or interpersonal talk are incredibly healthy depression treatments that are just some of the available psychosocial depression treatments that cognitive behavior therapists can offer to their patients, both actually prove to be able to produce fruitful and positive results even for just short-term sessions, around ten to twenty weeks are almost always, already enough to get a depression patient slowly begin their recovery towards a sound mental health.

Before getting started with depression medication, the depression patient must first get him or herself to a reputable doctor, get a diagnosis of which type of depression the patient is actually suffering from, may it be clinical depression, manic depression or what-have-you. It's best that you're sure what you're actually dealing with since there are various depression medications that are available in the market, you should make sure that you get the most appropriate one, the one that'll actually cure your depression illness.

There's actually a wide variety of anti-depressant depression medications available to help treat those who are suffering from depressive disorders. The more popular ones are those that are of the selective serotonin reuptake inhibitors or SSRIs variant then there are the tricyclics while the other popular variant is the monoamine oxidase inhibitors or MAOIs. These depression medications (the SSRIs variant as well as the other newer depression medication available in the market) actually to be a much safer alternative than the tricyclics, since they have fewer side-effects as opposed to the tricyclics depression medication variant.

How To Win Your War Against Depression

Sometimes, doctors actually find it more effective to mix up these depression medications, depending on the needs of the individual, the doctor might actually prescribed a variety of depression medication to help cure one's depression illness. Also the dosages of depression medication can actually be increased or lowered depending on what the doctor finds to be the most effective. However, when it comes to taking these depression medications, patients are highly advised to never mix up depression medications as well as pick out which dosages to take without consulting their doctors first.

Anti-anxiety or sedatives however, should never be mistaken as depression medication. Even though these anti-anxiety drugs are often prescribed along with depression medication, they don't actually help cure one's depression illness. Their mere purpose is to help calm one's nerves which is why depression medications are still needed to be taken by the depression patient.

There are actually some common side-effects from depression medication, usually coming from the tricyclic variety. Some people tend to not mind these side-effects from depression medication, however if it does become to much of a bother and may end up ruining one's ability to function properly, it's best to go immediately to your doctor and report the side-effects. Quite common side-effects from depression medication are the following:

Dry mouth: always having the irritating feeling of being hydrated, it's best to always have some (clean, drinking) water nearby so as to have something to drink whenever dry mouth occurs, chewing sugar free gum as well as brushing your teeth after every meal is also a good idea.

Constipation: cure such discomfort by eating and taking in a lot of fiber to help aid your digestion.

Blurry vision: another temporary side-effect, this one's quite easy to pass but if it proves to be too much of a bother, consult your doctor immediately.

Headaches: quite common with the newer kinds of depression medication, it's really not a big deal and will actually go away easily.

How To Win Your War Against Depression

Insomnia: first-time users may actually experience this depression medication side-effect but it usually just happens during the first few weeks of taking the depression medication, asking your doctor to lower the dosage of the depression medication may actually help you with this side-effect, as well as the time of day wherein you take your depression medication can actually have something to do with your sleeping problem.

Finding The Right Depression Treatment

Depression or prolonged sadness is actually quite common in the United States, around 9.5 percent of the American population actually suffers from this illness, however, not all of them get to be treated, thus, depression and its ill-effects continue to be a burden to some individuals. This illness may seem quite simple to treat but in reality, it takes more than a little cheering up to actually cure depression. Constant visits to a cognitive behavior therapist is a must as well as taking all the prescribed medicines that the doctor will ask the patient to take – none of these exactly come cheap, but the amount of suffering that a person is going through because of depression is enough reason already for others to start taking notice and face depression head on through the various depression treatments that are available today.

 Depression oftentimes can easily get in the way of an individual's daily activities and his or hers' normal functions, one's zest for life can quickly and easily dissipate due to depression. And in place of an individual's sunny disposition is more or less a person who hates his or herself, having no self-confidence, trying to isolate one's self from the world and basically just not caring about living any more. More so, a person suffering from depression isn't the only one who's going to suffer from this destructive illness, his or her loved ones are sure to follow suit. By seeing the individual grow through such rough patches, basically not caring about anything or anyone anymore, it's highly likely that not only will depression one's relationship with one's self but with his or her loved ones too. But this shouldn't really pose as such a problem since people who suffer from depression are actually lucky that there are all sorts of depression treatments that can be used to aid an individual through the course of having a sound mental health.

Depression treatment actually starts with the patient openly acknowledging his or her illness, by just being honest with one's self, it'll be a lot easier not only for the doctor but for the patient most of all, to actually cure depression and find an appropriate depression treatment for him or her.

From various medications (like Zoloft antidepressant depression treatment) to all sorts of psychotherapies promising to be the best depression treatment. The patient, as well as his or her family are sure to get the best, positive results from these depression treatments.

How To Win Your War Against Depression

Psychotherapy, a popular type of depression treatment actually includes short-term therapy sessions, usually from ten to twenty weeks promising to actually be able to make positive results for the depression patient. This type of depression treatment actually helps the individual by slowly making them to actually open up about their feelings, the root of their problems, more so, the root of their depression. Healthy verbal exchanges between the cognitive behavior therapist and the depression patient is great depression treatment that'll positively affect the depression patient by helping him or her discuss and talk about whatever they've been keeping inside.

Various medications that are available for depression treatment are actually great for helping the depression patient to regulate his or her mood swings, to actually help him or her sleep better and as well as be more pleasant towards others.

Facing Depression Head On

Always feeling under the weather? Always not in the mood to be around others and have a good time? If you're suffering from prolonged sadness for quite some time now, you should face these bouts of depression and get yourself diagnosed by a psychiatrist, they're doctors who can actually help you out with your problem.

Depression or prolonged sadness is actually quite common in the United States, around 9.5 percent of the American population actually suffer from this illness, however, not all of them get to be treated, thus, depression and its ill-effects continue to be a burden to some individuals. This illness may seem quite simple to treat but in reality, it takes more than a little cheering up to actually cure depression. Constant visits to a cognitive behavior therapist is a must as well as taking all the prescribed medicines that the doctor will ask the patient to take – none of these exactly come cheap, but the amount of suffering that a person is going through because of depression is enough reason already for others to start taking notice and face depression head on.

Depression oftentimes can easily get in the way of an individual's daily activities and his or her's normal functions, one's zest for life can quickly and easily dissipate due to depression. And in place of an individual's sunny disposition is more or less a person who hates his or herself, having no self-confidence, trying to isolate one's self from the world and basically just not caring about living any more. More so, a person suffering from depression isn't the only one who's going to suffer from this destructive illness, his or her loved ones are sure to follow suit. By seeing the individual grow through such rough patches, basically not caring about anything or anyone anymore, it's highly likely that not only will depression one's relationship with one's self but with his or her loved ones too.

Fortunately depression can now be cured, especially when diagnosed early, depressed individuals can actually be treated through therapy and medication, although it may be a bit costly, a person's good mental health is something that shouldn't be scrimped on. Cognitive behavioral talk or interpersonal talk are just some of the available psychosocial treatments that cognitive behavior therapists can offer to their patients, both actually prove to be able to produce fruitful and positive results.

How To Win Your War Against Depression

Still, people tend to not recognize depression even it's right before their eyes, being honest with one's self is key to being able to cure such an illness. Never overlook the various symptoms, depressed individuals oftentimes exhibit uncharacteristic behaviors such as suddenly lacking interest in one's hobbies (or other stuff that he or she usually enjoys), sleeps too much or actually aren't able to get some shut-eye, suddenly becoming anti-social, talks a lot about death or being a worthless person. There are actually a lot more other symptoms but in case these already fit in your category or of someone that you know of, go to a reputable psychiatrist at once in order to see if the depression is still at an early stage or not. From here you'll be able to assess how the treatments will actually go.

Depression shouldn't be something that people fear of, instead, people should just start taking charge of their lives and actually face this illness and fight it. Life is too beautiful a gift to waste and if one will spend the majority of his or her life just moping around about every single little thing then what kind of life would that be? Depression may not kill one's body but it'll certainly kills one's spirit if you'll let it. Don't be a victim.

Manic Depression

Manic depression is a disorder that's also called bipolar disorder or manic-depressive illness. It's a mood disorder, but it's one of extremes. The term manic depression comes from the word mania which refers to the extreme highs and lows someone with bipolar disorder experiences. Bipolar disorder does not get better on its own and must be treated. There are numerous medical research studies being conducted in the area of manic depression, but current treatments often include medication.

With depression, you experience mostly, if not only, low feelings. With manic depression you experience extreme moods ranging from the most euphoric to the deepest depression. During the euphoric stage, the person is very happy and high-strung. The attention span is short, sleep is difficult, and it's hard to concentrate. But one of the most distressing symptoms during this euphoric stage is the loss of good judgment and the desire to be reckless. A person during this stage may charge up all the credit cards, gamble all their money away or engage in risky business or sexual decisions.

During the depression stage, a person with manic depression will experience deep feelings of sadness and guilt. Life becomes hopeless and suicidal thoughts can begin. The person has little interest in any activities and may sleep a lot or very little.

Of course, everyone is different. The euphoric and depression highs and lows can be fairly mild in some cases, but the behavior during these periods can be devastating to a family. A manic depressive can cause great financial and interpersonal problem between family members. Unfortunately, people with manic depression can also experience mood swings within short periods of time.   It's even possible to experience both euphoric and depression at the same time.

There are many different things that can trigger episodes of manic depression. They include drug use and a traumatic experience such as a death in the family. There are various treatments used for bipolar disorder. One of the most common is prescription medications that stabilize moods or serve as antidepressants. Another common treatment is counseling sessions with a therapist. A therapist can assist a person with manic depression in identifying

How To Win Your War Against Depression

when euphoric or depression episodes are about to happen. The goal is to determine if there are certain things which cause the episodes to happen. There are other treatments, but those are the most common.

It's important to understand that manic depression is a serious disorder that needs medical attention. But even while under a doctor's care, you must make sure you take your medication regularly and become aware of what's happening to you emotionally and mentally. Though research seems to indicate this disorder occurs because of faulty neurotransmitters, it's not known for sure. Manic depression is a complicated problem that needs medical attention.

Natural Cure For Depression

Some people absolutely refuse to take prescriptions medications unless it's a matter of life and death. Instead, they prefer to try a natural cure for depression. There are many natural treatments that people have tried in an attempt to deal with depression. Whether they work has not been scientifically documented in some cases, while others are known to be beneficial.

A natural cure for depression is one that doesn't rely on prescription medications as a solution. Instead, you may decide to try an herb or supplement or make dietary changes. Other natural cures involve learning relaxation techniques or massages to relieve stress. Whatever natural cure for depression you decide to use, it's still important to keep your doctor informed. Depression is a serious illness and nothing to take lightly. Your doctor can help you monitor your progress while using natural treatment alternatives.

You have a choice for a natural cure for depression. Actually, most people use more than one method. One of the commonly used treatments is herbs and supplements. St. John's wort is considered to work as a natural antidepressant in cases of mild depression. It's an ancient perennial that's been used for centuries in alternative medicine treatments. One thing to always keep in mind is that herbs can interact with prescription medicines. That's a good reason why you should always make sure your doctor knows what you are taking as supplements.

Another natural cure for depression people try is taking vitamins and minerals. One of the symptoms of depression is a radical change in weight. When you aren't getting proper nutrition, the problem only worsens. Also depression affects concentration and some vitamins and minerals are considered to be mental aids. These include vitamin B and folic acid.

Yet another natural cure for depression is changing dietary habits. Turkey, for example, has an amino acid which assists the production of serotonin. Other foods include milk and potatoes. You can also eat foods high in omega-3 fatty acids such as soybeans and fish. All of these foods can aid with the brain's chemical production, insure you are getting proper nutrition and hopefully decrease depression.

How To Win Your War Against Depression

There are lots of other natural treatments for depression that people have tired including nerve stimulation. But one of the most popular is learning relaxation techniques which also may include massages. One of the causes of depression is an overload of stress. Relaxation methods teach you how to take control of anxious thoughts and turn them around. People who are anxious and depressed often make their situation worse just because they don't know how to calm themselves. There's no proof this is true, but it certainly cannot hurt.

If you want to avoid using medications or don't have time or money for traditional treatments for depression, you should investigate trying a natural cure for depression.

Postpartum Depression

Postpartum depression has been a disorder society has had a hard time accepting. After all, when you have a baby it should only bring great happiness to your life. Yet, being pregnant and having a baby is also a time when the body goes through enormous stress and hormones are produced in excess amounts. In most women this may cause some minor and unpredictable mood changes, but in others it's quite possible it creates postpartum depression.

Though hormones are the suspect, there's no definitive proof yet that hormones are the only culprit. Postpartum depression is a very serious disorder that affects women within weeks of giving birth. For some women, the depression begins after only a few days.

Postpartum depression becomes apparent when the new mother has difficulty accepting responsibility for the new infant. There may be lack of interest in the baby or quick irritation when the baby cries. Other symptoms of postpartum depression include the following.

• Unable to sleep
• Feelings of inadequacies
• Exhaustion
• Inability to cope with baby care
• Despondency

The interesting fact is that a woman go complete an entire pregnancy with no signs of anxiety, and then develop postpartum depression after birth. Some cases of postpartum depression are severe and include unexplained and frequent crying and even thoughts of suicide. The new mother has trouble functioning and can't seem to complete the smallest chores. Also, some women show lack of interest in the infant.

It's an unpleasant subject, but postpartum depression has been determined to be the cause of a mother injuring the infant or infant siblings. In the severest cases, postpartum depression can develop into a psychosis. A psychosis means the woman is probably hallucinating or has lost a grip on reality. In many of these cases brought to court, the new mother claims she heard voices telling her the baby or her other children must be killed.

How To Win Your War Against Depression

The only reason this is discussed is because it's important to understand that postpartum depression is very real and must be treated. Ignoring the disorder does not make it go away. Fortunately, there are treatments that work well. In most cases, medication is prescribed by the doctor.

If you suspect you, or someone you know has postpartum depression, you should see a doctor immediately. Most women will experience some mild depression after the birth of a baby due to shifting hormones or the realization this child is now a continual responsibility. Before a baby is born, women gets lots of concerned attention from family and friends. Once the baby comes, and the mother is doing fine, the attention stops and the work begins. But postpartum depression is a serious disorder that must be dealt with before symptoms worsen.

Psychotic Depression

Generally speaking, psychotic depression is as bad as depression can get. It's a form of major depression whereby you lose touch with reality. Unfortunately, tragedy can occur unless others know what's going on in your mind. Anyone who watches the news has seen mothers on trial for killing children because "God said she had to because they are possessed". In other sensational trials, the devil has "spoken" to people and told them to do unthinkable acts or violence.

Psychotic depression has several common symptoms. They include the following.

• Hearing voices
• Delusional thinking
• Hallucinating
• Paranoia
• Delusions

When you have psychotic depression, your reality is different from others. You may believe space aliens are talking to you on your cell phone. Or you think the voices you hear are telling you to harm yourself. Obviously, you should not try to treat this type of depression on your own. Treatment will probably require some hospitalization and most certainly medication.

There is a new type of medication being used in cases of severe depression. It's called atypical antipsychotic. They have worked in cases where SSRIs and tricyclics have not proven effective. This is good news for those with psychotic depression, because the often help those with the severest forms of depression. Unfortunately, they do have many possible side effects. A person taking one of these drugs must be monitored at all times. The side effects include the following.

• Facial tics
• Weight gain
• Movement problems
• Hypertension

How To Win Your War Against Depression

• Blurred vision

This is not a comprehensive list, but gives you a good idea of the kind of side effects people are experiencing as a result of using the atypical antipsychotics. Unfortunately, when a person is hallucinating or has become suicidal, the use of medications is necessary even with the unpleasant side effects. Psychotic depression is a very serious disorder that can't wait for the perfect treatment to be discovered. The good news is medical researchers are constantly looking for alternative treatments for psychotic depression.

Treatment for psychotic depression will be long and complicated. This is not something that can be handled easily which is why it must be treated by a doctor. When someone is psychotic, they cannot monitor their own treatment until they reach a certain level of mental wholeness.

If you or someone you know is experiencing any of the symptoms listed above, it's imperative you seek treatment from a doctor. Though it's a complicated disorder, it's treatable most of the time. The doctor will probably prescribe medication in addition to another therapy such as group therapy or cognitive therapy. No one needs to suffer with this disorder alone when there are so many ways to treat psychotic depression.

Signs of Depression

There are so many different signs of depression which means it sometimes continues until the indications form a pattern. But the sooner you recognize depression in yourself or someone else, the sooner you can get treatment. Depression needs to be treated whether it's mild or severe or anything in between the extremes. Depression doesn't disappear on its own and will only get worse.

There are some basic and common signs of depression. They include the following.

- No feelings of self worth or low self esteem
- Doesn't like to be around other people which can include family
- Doesn't anticipate doing anything including enjoyable events
- Lack of concentration
- Feelings of hopelessness
- Feeling sad all the time
- Suicidal thoughts
- Inability to make any decisions

A person can have one or more of these signs of depression. It's natural to feel sad for a few days or to have stressful days. It's normal to have some days when life may seem a little harder than you think it should be. Depression is something entirely different. It's not natural to feel you are worthless or that people in your life wouldn't miss you if you were to disappear. It's not normal to be sad for longer than two weeks while continuing to experience constant fatigue and lack of interest in anything around you.

The signs of depression can be very noticeable in many cases. Someone who is depressed may cry a lot for no apparent reason. In severe cases, a person may refuse to get out of bed. In milder cases, the person might be unable to make the simplest decision or constantly feels guilty about something. People with depression can have trouble functioning at work or at home.

How To Win Your War Against Depression

Other signs of depression may not be severe and are harder to identify. For example, you can experience depression triggered by an event such as a death in the family or loss of a job. It can be a real shock and not everyone is able to adjust well. You might still appear to function normally but the signs of depression are there. You might cry at the most unexpected times or begin a spiral into despondency that makes you unable to function eventually.

On the other hand, bipolar disorder has very obvious symptoms. While in a euphoric state, bizarre behavior such as making obviously foolish and harmful decision becomes apparent. While in a depressed state, the person feels hopeless and all the frenetic activity stops. This happens over and over again and can even happen within a day.

The key to identifying if someone is depressed is to watch for patterns or continual worsening of suspect symptoms.   If this goes on for longer than 2 weeks, you should get professional help for you or your friend or family member.

The Tell-Tale Symptoms Of Depression

People who may be suffering from depression or manic disorders actually exhibit or show each and every kind of symptom of depression that doctors will tell you that depressed people have. Sometimes it's actually quite easy to overlook such symptoms and not be able to help one's self or others who are suffering from depression for that matter.

There are actually a lot of symptoms of depression that depressed people may actually posses but they don't have to suffer from each and every one of them before you actually help them get diagnosed and be treated for this illness. Also, since symptoms of depression actually vary, the time of their "attacks" varies as well.

Here are some common examples of symptoms of depression:

Prolonged period of sadness or not feeling "up to it," people who are always feeling not in the mood, who'd rather mope around the house and feel sorry for one's self is the best example for this symptom of depression.

Feels hopeless, perennial pessimist: speaking of feeling sorry for one's self, another common symptom of depression is when a person actually feels like he/she has nothing to look forward to in his or her life. As for being the perennial pessimist, those who show this symptom of depression are usually very negative about things, again, the feeling of hopelessness comes in to mind.

Guilt-driven, loss of self-worth and helplessness: other symptoms of depression that can be easily seen on people who prefer to mope around all day long are these. Whenever a person feels so guilty over something, that actually makes one a very sad person who feels like he or she doesn't deserve to be happy. Thus, the loss of self-worth, if that person feels like he or she isn't worthy of being happy or enjoying one's self then that's clear tell-tale symptom of depression. Helplessness also contribute to being depressed, when assuming that things won't simply go your way, it's already a clear saying that you have absolutely no hope in your body at all.

How To Win Your War Against Depression

Isn't interested in finding or taking pleasure; just dropping the hobbies as well as the other things that one used to enjoy: this tell-tale symptom of depression just shows how depressed a person can be, if one is actually too sad to take pleasure even in the very things that one loves then that person is seriously lacking something, rather, that person might well have caught the depression bug.

Fatigue, always tired: people suffering from depression, since they've lost whatever interest in life that they may have had before are actually lacking of physical energy at all times, if one would prefer to just mope around, probably won't even eat not get enough sleep, a depressed person may well be on their way to not just a mental illness but depression can actually be terrible for one's physical health as well.

Having trouble concentrating, having bad memory and is indecisive: a person who is suffering from depression easily gives away this tell-tale symptom of depression. Wherein one's lack of interest with regards to the outside world or for just about anything for that matter can lead to that person's inability to lose track of things and actually not be able to remember things that happened or what other people said. Lack of interest actually makes depressed people very inattentive.

There are actually more symptoms of depression that can actually help you see if a person (or you) needs to be brought to the doctor to get some help when it comes to depression: lacking sleep, sleeping too much or waking up at wee hours of the morning are all symptoms of depression (if it happens on a daily basis), appetite loss as well as eating too much may show one's lack of enthusiasm for life. Be weary of sudden weight loss or weight gain in those around you. Being suicidal, talking about death, about wanting to die is another clear indication that that person is depressed. Being restless and irritable and physical symptoms that are usually brought about by poor mental health such as headaches, digestive disorders and various body pains.

Teen Depression

Sometimes teenagers can be hard to interpret because they have many normal ups and downs as they grow into adults. But teen depression is a growing problem as evidenced by the increasing number of teen suicides. It's also not unusual to hear parents of teenagers involved in violent acts in the schools say the teens had been depressed. But it's sometimes hard to differentiate between the normal emotional variability due to hormonal changes and true depression.

As parents of teenagers, it's important to watch for changes in behavior that don't make sense and seem to worsen as times go by. For example, teenagers that have always enjoyed being with friends and then suddenly stop socializing may be experiencing depression. Losing interest in activities is one of the major signs of depression. Teen depression may reveal itself in other ways too.

• Loss of interest in sports activities when sports have always been important

• Sudden drops in grades at school

• Change in eating habits such as loss of appetite or ravenous gorging

• Comments indicating low self-esteem

• Sudden fluctuations in moods

It would be nice if an adolescent would just tell a parent exactly what he or she is thinking and feeling, but that often doesn't happen. Instead the parents have to be acutely aware of unusual behavior that indicates something's not right in their child's life.

There are ongoing medical studies trying to find physical reasons for teen depression. There has been a correlation found between obesity and depression. That only makes sense when you consider the symptoms of depression in children. For example, an obese child can have feelings of low self worth due to peer taunting. Teenagers who are depressed may eat a lot of "comfort food" seeking solace for their feelings of isolation. Teenagers can also be

How To Win Your War Against Depression

experiencing problems at school and not be telling the parents at home. As a parent you think things are going well only to discover there's been an ongoing problem between students or student and teacher.

Adolescents can be very sensitive human beings. The teenage years are formative years, and when problems in socialization occur, it can be very demoralizing. In addition, sudden mood swings can also indicate there's another problem in the teen's life. If a teenager is being abused physically or sexually, teen depression can be the response.

Identifying teen depression can be difficult, but never impossible. When you suspect your child may be experiencing teen depression, you should try to talk to the child first. If the adolescent won't talk to you then professional therapy may be in order. It's important that some kind of treatment be instituted, because the lack of self esteem can be devastating. Depression deepens and doesn't just disappear once he or she reaches adulthood. Your teenager can become a depressed adult next.

Of course, one of the best treatments you can give your child is always lots of love!

Treatments For Depression

There are many treatments for depression and usually more than one is used at a time. The most common treatments today include the following.

• Cognitive therapy
• Group therapy
• Medication
• Behavioral therapy
• Interpersonal therapy

Most of the treatments for depression include keeping a journal as a first step and even an activity log when the depression is severe enough to prevent you from completing critical activities. A log can be an important tool for both you and/or your therapist in order to identify the triggers of depression. It can also be a good way to get your life back on track.

One of the benefits of using journals and logs in the treatments for depression is that it forces you to undertake an activity to improve your life. This can be very important when depression has interfered with your ability to think or function normally. For example, if you keep a log of what you're feeling and of your thoughts, it becomes easier to identify the negative thinking that spirals out of control. A journal can reveal things such as feelings of failure or anxiety. With the identification of the thoughts, a therapist can then help you seek the cause of the lack of self esteem.

An activity log is a useful log during any of the treatments for depression for keeping track of what must be done in your life to keep it on track. People with depression often decide they don't care anymore about any one or any thing. Unfortunately, this can have dire consequences if you don't pay bills or deposit money in your bank account. Some people with depression don't just neglect themselves either. They neglect important tasks such as picking up the kids at school. The can even decide eating is too much trouble. That's why some people with depression can have sudden and severe weight loss.

When people get depressed, the mind focuses on dark and deep thoughts that are usually self-critical. If you tell yourself you're unable to do anything right, the next logical thought is: why

How To Win Your War Against Depression

try? That is how depression works. It gets deeper and deeper if left untreated. Except for medication, the treatments for depression assist people with changing their thought patterns so they see themselves as capable and positive.

It's hard for someone who's never had depression to understand how deep the mental hole can get. When you keep a journal and activity log, you can learn to set simple goals that are easy to meet. The slow decline into the black hole is reversed so you can begin the upward climb to the light. It's done one step at a time. There's no instant cure for depression. Even medication takes time to work.

Understanding Zoloft Depression Better

Always feeling under the weather? Always not in the mood to be around others and have a good time? If you're suffering from prolonged sadness for quite some time now, you should face these bouts of depression and get yourself diagnosed by a psychiatrist, they're doctors who can actually help you out with your problem. Also, with the introduction of Zoloft depression, the number one, most-prescribed medicine for depression treatment, the problems concerning depression can easily be gone.

Depression or prolonged sadness is actually quite common in the United States, around 9.5 percent of the American population actually suffer from this illness, however, not all of them get to be treated, thus, depression and its ill-effects continue to be a burden to some individuals. This illness may seem quite simple to treat but in reality, it takes more than a little cheering up to actually cure depression. Constant visits to a cognitive behavior therapist is a must as well as taking all the prescribed medicines that the doctor will ask the patient to take – none of these exactly come cheap, but the amount of suffering that a person is going through because of depression is enough reason already for others to start taking notice and face depression head on. Here's where Zoloft depression actually steps in, proven to be a safe and very effective treatment for various types of depression as well as anxiety, Zoloft depression has actually been around for around 12 years. Patients have been proven to respond well to treatments from Zoloft depression while doctors favor Zoloft depression's availability in various strengths, this way, someone who's suffering from depression doesn't have to settle for something else just cause they don't have the right dosage available, with Zoloft depression, it's hard to not get the right dosage for you.

In a nutshell, Zoloft depression is actually a type of antidepressant which is known to people as "selective serotonin reuptake inhibitor" or SSRI. It's well-known to be a good treatment for patients over the age of eighteen that are being treated for the following: depression, posttraumatic disorder or PTSD, social anxiety disorder, panic disorder, premenstrual dysphoric disorder or PMDD and obsessive-compulsive disorder or OCD.

Some commonly asked questions about Zoloft depression are the following:

How To Win Your War Against Depression

How long does it take before the effect of Zoloft depression actually kicks in?

How important is it to follow the doctor's prescription for Zoloft depression?

To be frank, Zoloft depression is actually not for everyone, those patients who are taking pimozide or MAOIs are strictly discouraged from using Zoloft depression. Various side effects can stem from actually using Zoloft depression such as: diarrhea, nausea, sleepiness/insomnia, dry mouth and sexual side effects. Although according to studies, a lot of people actually didn't care about the side effects and still opted to continue on taking Zoloft depression.

Some good points to consider though is that Zoloft depression is actually in no way addicting unlike other medication and it is not in any way, can be associated with weight gain.

Since Zoloft depression actually comes in various dosages (25mg, 50mg and 100mg tablets), it is definitely best to consult your doctor first before taking any Zoloft depression tablet. This is one of the main reasons why Zoloft depression was actually created in various dosages, since each person is unique, one's need for Zoloft depression may actually differ from the other and that is why we need professional doctors to assess how much or how little of Zoloft depression does one actually need. Self medication has always been a problem of doctors since their patients usually just end up in worse state than usual whenever they self-medicate and conduct their own diagnosis.

Depending on a person's body makeup or ability to respond to treatments as well as one's willingness to actually help him or herself get better, the effects of Zoloft depression can be felt in as early as 2 weeks, just continue on following the doctors prescriptions as well as showing up for every therapy session, Zoloft depression will seriously work for you.

How To Win Your War Against Depression

This Product Is Brought To You By

DAVID A OSEI